# HEALTH HOROSCOPE

*Caring for the stars of the zodiac signs*

Alex Magic

# CONTENTS

# PREFACE

Today's world requires us to carefully plan our affairs, and the violation of these plans entails unpleasant consequences: disruption of schedules, lost profits, missing important events and even interruption of vacation. Therefore, taking care of your own health is the responsibility of a modern person. Standard health prevention is always present in the daily routine of successful people - it can be both sports and conditioning. But it is very difficult to predict what exactly awaits us in the near future and, therefore, to take appropriate measures to prevent dangers. Health can be shattered by many factors, from the occasional draft and infection to poor-quality food and a bad fall.

It is impossible to avoid all this, unless, of course, you know where to "lay the straws." Someone doused with cold water every day, but stumbled on the subway and got dislocated or, for example, engaged in oriental meditations, but seasonal allergies suddenly spoil the pleasure of relaxation. Knowing the future, even the most probable one, would simplify our plans and expectations, allowing some of our worries to be diverted to other areas of life. Fortunately, the stars, united in key constellations, called the zodiacal, can communicate what awaits us in the near future. One of the oldest sciences comes to our aid.

# HEALTH HOROSCOPE

Today's world requires us to carefully plan our affairs, and the violation of these plans entails unpleasant consequences: disruption of schedules, lost profits, missing important events and even interruption of vacation. Therefore, taking care of your own health is the responsibility of a modern person. Standard health prevention is always present in the daily routine of successful people - it can be both sports and conditioning. But it is very difficult to predict what exactly awaits us in the near future and, therefore, to take appropriate measures to prevent dangers. Health can be shattered by many factors, from the occasional draft and infection to poor-quality food and a bad fall.

It is impossible to avoid all this, unless, of course, you know where to "lay the straws." Someone doused with cold water every day, but stumbled on the subway and got dislocated or, for example, engaged in oriental meditations, but seasonal allergies suddenly spoil the pleasure of relaxation. Knowing the future, even the most probable one, would simplify our plans and expectations, allowing some of our worries to be diverted to other areas of life. Fortunately, the stars, united in key constellations, called the zodiacal, can communicate what awaits us in the near future. One of the oldest sciences comes to our aid.

# HEALTH HOROSCOPE: ARIES

Representatives of the sign Aries from early childhood are the owners of good health. These are energetic and active people, characterized by increased endurance. Thanks to a positive attitude, Aries quickly cope with troubles and try not to get hung up on illnesses. In most cases, they themselves become the culprits of health problems. Representatives of the fire element often work for wear and tear and devote little time to rest and sleep, considering it a useless waste of time. Neglecting your body leads to the acquisition of chronic diseases and increased irritability. In addition, the health horoscope warns Aries of a high tendency to various injuries, from which the head most often suffers.

## *Aries man health horoscope*

Aries men are distinguished by good health and a youthful appearance, which they are able to maintain until old age. Overweight people are rarely found among the representatives of the fire element. Thanks to their active lifestyle and passion for sports, they always stay in good physical shape. The flip side of increased energy is overwork and insomnia, which Aries men treat quite normally and do not consider it a problem. They practically do not notice the onset of the disease and ignore the first symptoms. Men born under this sign rarely seek help from doctors, preferring to endure the disease on their feet.

Representatives of the fire element do not like to listen to the opinion of professionals, believing that they know better how to cope with the disease. Such stubbornness often leads to various complications, which become much more difficult to cope with. The list of typical Aries diseases includes cerebrovascular accident, brain inflammation, neuralgia, migraine. Men born under this sign often suffer from high blood pressure, sore throat, gum infection, tooth decay, and abscesses.

Aries men should pay attention to their eye health, especially in old age. Increased nervous excitability can cause heart attack and stroke. In addition, representatives of the fire element are often prone to colds, which can become chronic. The Aries health horoscope recommends avoiding dangerous situations, as there is a high risk of serious injury. They also should not get carried away with alcoholic beverages and lean on caffeine, because of the high probability of developing addiction.

## *Aries woman health horoscope*

Aries women are the owners of strong immunity, which they can boast of even in old age. Since childhood, the representatives of this sign show great activity and energy. These are real fidgets, interested in all things in the world. Despite this, Aries women do not like to play sports. They are prone to fatty and unhealthy foods, and therefore can fight extra pounds throughout their lives.

Aries women often neglect the treatment of emerging diseases. This approach usually leads to the acquisition of chronic ailments that are not easy to get rid of. Despite excellent health, representatives of the fire element often suffer from overwork. Increased impulsivity and lack of patience often lead to problems with blood pressure. In addition, the irascibility of this sign leads to migraines and nerves. Improper nutrition affects the work of the gastrointestinal tract. This is expressed in frequent frustration, constipation, vomiting and nausea.

The health horoscope for Aries advises the fair sex to follow a diet, regularly arrange fasting days and not abuse flour products. Also, do not neglect the prevention of colds and infectious diseases. In the winter season, more attention should be paid to the health of the genitourinary system. There is a risk of kidney and bladder problems.

## Good and bad habits

Aries are very sociable and sociable people who are not afraid to make new acquaintances. A distinctive feature of their character is stubbornness. She can both become a helper in life and destroy relationships with friends and relatives. People born under this sign strive to be leaders and do not admit their mistakes. They often manifest themselves as real selfish. Despite this, representatives of the fire element most often make the best friends. They will come to the aid of a person who is not indifferent to them more than once and will not demand anything in return.

Aries are overwhelmed with emotions. Alcohol helps them to calm down and come to balance, which they can drink in large quantities, and moreover, alone. Also, representatives of this sign will not give up good tobacco. Aries' bad habits can easily be attributed to the abuse of sweets: sugar saves them from stressful situations and during periods of nervous tension. However, Aries themselves never admit to the presence of addiction, trying to turn their weaknesses into a joke. Only close people who have paid attention to the problem in time will be able to find a way out of this situation.

## Diseases and dangers, vulnerabilities

Despite their good health, Aries can suffer from a wide variety of diseases. They are mainly subject to head diseases. These include spasms of the cerebral vessels, migraines, neuralgia of the facial nerves, memory impairments, dizziness and nervous exhaustion. Representatives of this sign are often not able to correctly calculate their strengths, which is why they literally work until they lose consciousness. They often deal with insomnia and depression, which manifests itself in the form of fear of premature death and incurable diseases.

For people born under this sign, diseases such as fever, hypertension, internal hemorrhage are characteristic. In older age, Aries can face stroke and heart attack. Throughout their lives, they are haunted by chronic colds with pronounced symptoms such as high fever, cough, chills, dizziness. Representatives of the fire element suffer from problems with the digestive system. They are characterized by diseases such as stomach ulcers, constipation and gastritis. Due to the high pain threshold, Aries do not notice the first symptoms of many diseases. For representatives of this sign, the best way out will be a regular medical examination, which will help to identify the disease at an early stage.

## Diet recommendations

Representatives of the Aries sign must adhere to a balanced diet. The Aries diet should exclude fatty foods that can cause blockage of blood vessels in the brain. The diet of representatives of the fire element must contain fermented milk products, vegetables, cereals and cereals, fruits, nuts. An unhealthy diet can slow down your reaction time and cause stomach problems. You can eat lean meat no more than 2-3 times a week. The lack of protein foods can be easily compensated for with seafood, dairy products and all kinds of cereals.

Aries' diet must necessarily contain foods rich in vitamin C. First of all, these are citrus fruits, for example, oranges and lemons, as well as bananas and apples. In winter, the menu should include dried fruits, cranberries, lingonberries, viburnum. Sauerkraut can be a great source of vitamins for Aries. It is better for representatives of this sign to exclude strong coffee from their diet. The best substitute for it would be herbal tea made from rose hips, sea buckthorn, hawthorn, raspberries and hibiscus. Brain-friendly foods rich in potassium phosphate include cucumbers, tomatoes, radishes, onions, apples, spinach, carrots, beets, and cauliflower.

## Fitness and sports, outdoor activities

Aries of both sexes are incredibly active and energetic people. They can achieve immense success in any sport if they wish. In most cases, people born under this sign prefer team-based physical activity. Thanks to their leadership qualities, they will be able to achieve serious success in football, hockey, basketball, volleyball. Fitness horoscope for Aries advises people of the fire element to take a closer look at martial arts, in which they have high chances of winning. Representatives of this sign show excellent results in speed skating and all types of athletics. They love speed, so they often prefer car racing.

Aries are lovers of risk and excitement. For them, any kind of extreme sport will be the ideal choice, be it rock climbing, shooting or boxing. Less active representatives of this sign can show their intellectual abilities in such sports games as chess. Aries perform well in figure skating, gymnastics, swimming, tennis and fencing. However, long-distance running is not for them, endurance is not the same. Engaging in any sport, Aries should avoid traumatic situations and especially protect their head from blows. In the case of neglect, there is a high chance of bone breakage and joint dislocation.

## How to maintain and improve health

First of all, Aries should avoid overwork, which is the reason for subsequent well-being problems. The decline in vitality affects the work of all systems of the body, which is why you have to spend an internal reserve, which sooner or later comes to an end. The horoscope advises the representatives of this sign to maintain a healthy lifestyle and not neglect physical exercise. Exercising regularly will help prevent premature aging and keep the body in good shape.

Alcoholic drinks are extremely contraindicated for Aries. They can cause serious addiction, which will be difficult for the representatives of this sign to get rid of. In addition, irreparable harm to health can be caused by regular coffee, which does not in the best way affect the already energetic Aries. It is advisable to avoid stressful situations and not neglect outdoor recreation. The oral cavity requires increased attention. Regular prevention can help prevent tooth decay and gum disease.

# HEALTH HOROSCOPE: TAURUS

Outwardly, people born under the sign of Taurus give the impression of calm and balanced personalities, so they rarely suffer from serious nervous disorders. Since childhood, they can boast of excellent health, however, they also have their own weaknesses. Despite their excellent immunity, diseases sometimes overwhelm them. If this happens, the disease will be long-term with a high probability of becoming chronic. This is aggravated by the fact that Taurus are not big fans of going to doctors. According to the health horoscope, another serious problem that representatives of the elements of the earth can meet is overweight. They often struggle with the hated pounds throughout their lives.

## *Taurus man health horoscope*

Taurus men are in good health from an early age. They have strong immunity, thanks to which diseases do not often overcome them. However, if the illness strikes them, they can not expect a quick recovery. The course of the disease is complicated by the fact that representatives of the elements of the earth do not like to seek help from a doctor. They will delay until the last moment, when the disease has already become severe. At the same time, Taurus men will never neglect medical recommendations and will follow all the prescriptions to the last point. All the inconveniences during the treatment process are borne by them courageously and without whims.

Despite the severe course of disease, Taurus have huge internal reserves. Thanks to them, the recovery process is extremely fast and soon the representatives of this sign will be full of strength and energy. The most vulnerable organs in Taurus are the throat, hearing organs, lymphatic system and gastrointestinal tract. People born under this sign often suffer from a slow metabolism and related illnesses. Taurus often have ailments such as gastritis, constipation and diabetes mellitus. Colds and infectious diseases are common for them.

The health horoscope for Taurus advises them not to abuse alcohol and not indulge their own weaknesses. Taurus men have an increased tendency to addiction to alcohol and tobacco products, which negatively affects the state of their body. Representatives of this sign need to instill from childhood a love of exercise and healthy eating, as they have an increased tendency to overeating and laziness.

## *Taurus woman health horoscope*

Taurus women are individuals with excellent health. However, due to their unwillingness to take care of him, they often suffer from various diseases. Taurus are prone to a variety of excesses in food and have more than one bad habit. In this regard, they devote most of their lives to the fight against extra pounds. In many cases, their dislike for doctors and unwillingness to seek help turns into the acquisition of chronic ailments, which will subsequently be difficult to get rid of.

The Taurus health horoscope says that most often the fair sex is faced with diseases of the throat, brain, nervous system, digestive system, liver, circulatory system and thyroid gland. Also among the characteristic ailments one can find diseases of the respiratory and genitourinary systems, and in particular of the kidneys. A frequent guest is colds and infectious diseases, which sometimes become chronic.

Taurus women are advised to avoid stress and observe the daily routine. Otherwise, there is a high chance of getting depression and insomnia. Representatives of this sign need to be in the fresh air as much as possible and in no case neglect physical activity. Astrologers advise people born under this sign to avoid drafts and crowded places during the height of infectious diseases.

## Good and bad habits

Unlike representatives of other signs, Taurus try to adhere to a healthy lifestyle, as they are well aware of their weaknesses. Everyone can envy their willpower. They easily get rid of addictions, intuitively grasping the moment when to stop. Representatives of the elements of the earth do not differ in the speed of reaction and generally seem to be too slow from the outside. However, they approach all matters with thoroughness, thanks to which they often cope with the tasks set much better than others.

The most serious bad habits of Taurus are their great tendency to overeat. They are truly addicted to various sweets and junk food. Taurus is unlikely to be able to keep from an extra piece, which often has serious negative consequences for their health. Because of their love of overeating, representatives of this sign often suffer from excess weight. Many Taurus throughout their lives try to get rid of unnecessary pounds, which is an overwhelming task for many of them. All this is aggravated by their dislike of physical activity and unwillingness to work on themselves.

## Diseases and dangers, vulnerabilities

Thanks to excellent immunity, Taurus rarely get sick, but diseases are often severe and protracted. The health horoscope warns the representatives of this sign that in many cases, ailments overwhelm them suddenly. Often, the onset of the disease is disguised as ordinary fatigue, which is why Taurus in most situations misses the moment of the onset of illness. In many ways, people born under this sign are themselves to blame for the formation of sores, since they are irresponsible in their state of health. Usually, the throat and hearing organs suffer from the disorder of Taurus.

For representatives of the elements of the earth, diseases such as tonsillitis, bronchial asthma and diphtheria are characteristic. Frequent guests for Taurus are diseases of the organs of the genitourinary and reproductive systems. Often, people born under this sign suffer from a violation of the endocrine glands and renal failure. Excessive love of fatty foods can lead to intestinal colic, poisoning and skin problems. Excessive physical activity does not reflect in the best way on the condition of the lower limbs. Overstrain is also a common cause of osteochondrosis in Taurus.

## Diet recommendations

The diet for Taurus should not contain a large amount of sugar, starch and fats, since many representatives of the sign have been fighting obesity all their lives. They should eat a balanced diet and not neglect moderate physical activity in order not to gain excess weight. In the food that Taurus eat, sodium sulfate must be present. It can be found in foods such as beets, spinach, horseradish, cauliflower, cucumbers, pumpkin, onions, cranberries, and nuts. Celery can help prevent overeating. Fermented milk products have a positive effect on the intestinal microflora.

The Taurus menu must include foods that help the proper functioning of the thyroid gland. These include foods high in iodine, such as fish, seaweed, eggs, beans, fresh fruit, and salad. It is useful for Taurus from time to time to arrange fasting days and consume as much liquid as possible. At an older age, they are not recommended to get carried away with protein foods and reduce meat consumption to 2-3 times a week. Astrologers advise giving preference to lean beef, lean chicken and various seafood.

## *Fitness and sports, outdoor activities*

By their nature, representatives of the elements of the earth are calm and unhurried individuals. Fitness horoscope for Taurus recommends people born under this sign to choose a sports discipline that would suit their temperament. In most cases, Taurus are excellent at showing their talents in figure skating, speed skating and swimming. Due to their high endurance, Taurus makes excellent long-distance runners. Representatives of the elements of the earth do not like to take risks, as a result of which extreme sports are not suitable for them.

Good abilities are shown in team sports such as football or hockey. Weightlifting and bodybuilding allows Taurus to show their strength and endurance, in which they reach solid heights. They are good at arm wrestling and lifting. The main obstacle to conquering sports peaks for people born under this sign is their own laziness. To achieve high results, Taurus needs to accustom themselves to physical activity from childhood and choose only the discipline to which they really have a soul.

## *How to maintain and improve health*

The main source of most of Taurus' problems is their pessimistic thoughts. Representatives of this sign tend to fall into depression and assume a worse outcome. It is important for them to receive as much positive emotions as possible and in no case indulge in despondency. To maintain their well-being, astrologers recommend that they acquire a pleasant hobby that would distract them from their daily routine. Overeating negatively affects the health of Taurus. Representatives of the elements of the earth who are prone to overweight should reduce the amount of calories consumed and in no case abuse junk food. Also, do not lean on alcohol and tobacco.

Daily walks in the fresh air and regular physical activity will have a positive effect. With their help, they will not only be able to keep weight under control, but also receive a dose of positive emotions. Along with this, astrologers do not advise to heavily load the back and legs, as there is a risk of getting stretched and getting osteochondrosis. There is no need to make sudden movements or immediately start intense training. This can negatively affect the functioning of the heart. A sedentary lifestyle is also contraindicated in Taurus due to the increased likelihood of vascular occlusion and circulatory problems.

# HEALTH HOROSCOPE: GEMINI

Gemini are vivid representatives of the air element, which explains their incredible mobility and flexibility of perception of the world around them. The heavenly patron of this sign, Mercury, gave his wards the ability to adapt to any situation. The health horoscope for Gemini is ambiguous, it is determined by the person's lifestyle, his mood in certain life periods. The astral energy of this sign most of all affects the communication functions of the body - speech, the network of capillaries, the nervous system, the synchronization of the activity of organs and supporting processes. Being the fastest planet in the solar system, Mercury gives Gemini a high pace of life, which creates a significant load on the brain, the health of the central nervous system, and the small intestine. The Gemini health horoscope promises good health if you avoid brain strain. The danger is that the representatives of this sign "are in a hurry to live and in a hurry to feel." Striving for constant changes, self-improvement with vaguely formulated spiritual needs, can lead to frequent ailments and internal emptiness. The horoscope identifies three areas of risk - the respiratory system, digestion, and psyche.

## *Gemini man health horoscope*

It is difficult for a Gemini man to boast of good health. Having been ill in childhood with bronchitis, pharyngitis, not counting regular colds and viral diseases, the representative of this sign chooses one of two tactics towards adulthood: either he stops paying attention to ailments, periodic headaches, other signals of his body, or falls into a hypochondriacal state, passes countless examinations, looking for symptoms of various diseases. This behavior is typical of Gemini's dual nature, but both options are equally dangerous. The principle of "golden mean" will help to maintain health at an appropriate level. The Gemini man is not distinguished by a sense of increased responsibility - this character trait also extends to the attitude towards his own health.

However, it cannot be said that the health of a Gemini man cannot be good. The active influence of Mercury makes it easy to adjust any areas of life, if the situation requires it. Until the age of 30, this sign of the zodiac does not feel special health problems. In the future, if he does not ignore the signals of the body, but takes preventive measures to maintain health, the horoscope promises excellent health, right up to old age. The health of the nervous system deserves special attention during this period. The desire to assert oneself in life, to receive everything at once, is associated with great emotional overload. The horoscope advises to alternate active activity and rest - this is not a slowdown on the path to success, but providing yourself with additional energy.

After 40 years, the horoscope advises Gemini men to reconsider the food culture. During this life period, the health of the gastrointestinal tract becomes the most vulnerable. It is better to give up snacks, quick meals, junk food - it's time to include the rule in your lifestyle: "war is war, and lunch is on schedule." Another caveat in the health horoscope is attention to blood pressure. Hypertension can provoke vasoconstriction, disrupt blood circulation, which is extremely undesirable - metabolic processes in the Gemini's body occur faster than in representatives of other signs, the transportation of nutrients to the organs should occur without interruption. The horoscope warns: signals such as regular headache, tinnitus, aching extremities should be immediately heard and communicated to the doctor.

# *Gemini woman health horoscope*

The Gemini woman is a changeable nature. It is difficult to determine her desires not only for others, but also for herself. For an hour of communication with this attractive person, you can contemplate the full range of her inherent emotions. At the same time, she treats her health more responsibly than her male stellar counterpart. The health horoscope is favorable, subject to timely medical examination and resistance to bad habits. Risk areas - psyche and nervous system. The high emotionality of this sign creates strong mood swings, and sensual "swing" can bring the psyche to threatening states.

The health horoscope warns of the need to learn to control your emotional states. Even at the age of 20, it is advisable to practice meditation exercises. The purposeful and energetic Gemini woman amazes those around her with a variety of desires and plans. Moreover, the implementation of all of them occurs simultaneously. If there is a person nearby who can put the puzzles of her brain into a single picture, there is no need to worry about her health.

After 43 years, the horoscope advises Gemini women to pay attention to the respiratory organs. This airy person may literally lack air. The more she learns to manage her emotions before this age, the less likely she is to develop respiratory diseases. The key word here is to manage, if emotions are simply suppressed, health problems can worsen. By the age of 46, the representatives of this sign become more balanced, which allows their body to function relatively calmly. The horoscope advises to include in your life schedule hiking, swimming, sightseeing trips, reading books.

# *Good and bad habits*

Almost all of Gemini's health problems are related to nerves and incorrect mental attitudes. Representatives of this zodiac sign are prone to various phobias and stress. Gemini's bad habits are due to a low sense of responsibility. The first place in the rating of bad qualities is occupied by inattention and talkativeness. Another favorite pastime is to quit the job at the slightest difficulty. The horoscope advises this sign to learn to listen to the opponent in silence, not to run away from difficulties.

Representatives of this sign rarely become alcoholics, but they often become heavy smokers, although they are well aware that inner balance can be achieved in other ways. The useful habits of Gemini include their absolute independence from the opinions of others, high communication skills, curiosity, and the desire for self-improvement.

## *Diseases and dangers, vulnerabilities*

The most vulnerable point of Gemini's health horoscope is the nervous system. Respiratory organs, speech function and upper limbs are at risk, in the context of circulatory disorders in this zone. Most often, this sign is overtaken by diseases such as neurasthenia, psychosis, nervous breakdown, neuralgia, arthritis, bronchial asthma, speech disorders (lisp, stuttering, burr). From birth, Gemini have good immunity, but for it to manifest and work in full force, certain conditions are necessary.

Little Gemini needs a calm and welcoming atmosphere. If there are scandals, swearing, a totalitarian approach to raising a child in a family, an already unbalanced child will be "lost" in a whirlpool of emotions, acquiring various diseases and phobias. An important condition for well-being, the horoscope determines the clear regulation of the lifestyle: the mode of work and rest, the priority of goals, the sequence of actions, a healthy diet. Compliance with these conditions at all stages of life will allow Gemini to maintain health and enjoy the splendor of the world around them with their characteristic curiosity.

## Diet recommendations

The element of air has endowed this sign with incredible mobility. Being in constant movement, the representatives of this sign hardly focus on one issue - they strive to solve everything at once. At the same time, a vague idea that the result of such actions will also be uncertain can slow down their run through life. Moderation is very difficult for Gemini - this applies to relationships with people, and career, and nutrition. Representatives of this sign may at one moment decide to become vegetarians, adhere to this position for a long time, and then move to the category of meat eaters, become adherents of a raw food diet. The horoscope warns that such experiments can be detrimental to health.

The health horoscope advises adhering to an individually tailored diet. The diet must include low-fat varieties of meat and fish, cheeses, seafood, cereals, peaches, grapes, olives, zucchini - the trace elements contained in these products help to normalize the activity of the nervous system, strengthen immunity. The diet for Gemini should not contain strong tea and coffee, sweets, alcoholic beverages, animal fats - these products have a stimulating effect on the unstable nervous system of this zodiac sign.

## Fitness and sports, outdoor activities

From early childhood, Gemini run, jump, dive, deftly get into the most inaccessible places - the internal motor does not allow them to sit still. They are not afraid of either height or depth. Sport for them is both pleasure and an obligatory component of life. Fitness horoscope for Gemini advises to pay attention to such sports as tennis, fencing, biathlon, cycling, skiing. Trap shooting and sports knife throwing will be useful for psychological relief.

Gemini love to travel. New places, people, impressions satisfy their inner desire for constant movement. This sign does not accept measured sightseeing tours. Representatives of this sign will get real pleasure climbing mountain peaks, overcoming stormy rivers by kayak, and a tourist trip to the Far North will leave unforgettable impressions in their souls for many years.

## *How to maintain and improve health*

Possessing by nature strong immunity and good health, careless Gemini are able to squander this resource at the very beginning of their life. The first advice on maintaining and strengthening health, the horoscope addresses the parents of little Gemini: a calm, friendly atmosphere in the family, a strict, balanced diet, an established daily routine, systematic classes in sports sections - they will teach discipline, form the ability to organize their living space, teach to determine priority goals and objectives.

Adult Gemini are encouraged to adhere to the same principles. It is important to realize the duality of your nature, to correct your behavior, realizing that the habit of rushing from side to side is nothing more than a character trait. To reduce the impact on health of stressful situations, the horoscope recommends that naturally talented Gemini as a hobby to do art: music, painting, handicrafts, modeling - they are able to balance the unstable energy field of this sign, increase vitality, and strengthen mental health.

# HEALTH HOROSCOPE: CANCER

Cancer is one of the most unusual representatives of the zodiacal circle, a representative of the element of Water. His patron saint is the Moon, changeable and mysterious. Cancer depends on the phases of the satellite of the Earth, its mood often fluctuates, changes, behavior seems unpredictable and strange. But the representative of the water sign is not at all melancholic, but on the contrary, he is optimistic, loves to communicate, has a deep mind and a good sense of humor. Outwardly, this person seems balanced, calm, but hides within himself worries and fears. This is a very impressionable and sensitive nature, however, positive emotions, joyful events can at one moment improve the physical condition of the sign. The health horoscope for Cancer is not always favorable and largely depends on the mood of the person, his lifestyle.

## *Cancer man health horoscope*

The Cancer man is not in good health. By nature, people of this sign have a weak metabolism and circulation of fluid in the body. The head, skin, gastrointestinal tract, kidneys, bladder, and nervous system are vulnerable. This sign requires constant monitoring of the state of health, a positive attitude, a positive environment. Men of the water element are hardworking, they can make a career and achieve material wealth for themselves and their families. In addition, they are thrifty, do not waste money on their whims. But often they take on too many responsibilities that they cannot afford. The ability to work of the representatives of this sign depends on their well-being, they should correctly calculate their strength and not forget to take care of themselves.

This does not mean that a Cancer man cannot have good health. With an optimistic attitude, an active lifestyle, sports activities and a diet, the life of a representative of this sign promises to be long and fruitful. Monitoring the state of health, timely treatment are especially necessary after 40 years. It is impossible to withdraw into oneself, succumb to depression, rotate in the society of "whiners" who are fixated on talking about diseases. For a suspicious watermark, this is unacceptable. After hearing a story about death, severe illness or improper treatment, an impressionable Cancer can fall ill himself and go to bed for a long time. You should also avoid injuries, scratches that do not heal for a long time, cause physical suffering.

According to the health horoscope, the well-being of a Cancer man can be influenced by various phases of the moon, which either bring a surge of strength, or, on the contrary, take vital energy. Representatives of this sign feel best at home, in the family, in the most secluded and safe place. This is not surprising, because Cancer is one of the most loyal to the family of signs. This is a loving husband, a wonderful father who works for the sake of family values, brings every grain of grain to children, helps in building a cozy nest. Therefore, family representatives of the sign, with the support of loved ones, have the opportunity to live a long time without having serious health problems.

## Cancer woman health horoscope

A gentle and outwardly calm Cancer woman also feels best at home. This sensitive lady hides fears and anxieties inside, while maintaining external calm. Experiences can lead to the onset of illness, melancholy, depression. The health horoscope warns of the need to monitor nutrition, work and rest. If a woman devotes herself entirely to family responsibilities, forgetting about herself, then she can overwork and go to bed. She is a wonderful housewife, wife and mother who must be protected and cherished.

The representative of the water element is very impressionable, she absolutely does not tolerate criticism, rudeness and inattention. A vulnerable woman must constantly hear words of approval, support, which she needs more than others. Kind words, compliments, any manifestation of love will make her happy, prevent illness, nervous breakdowns. Family members must remember this in order to maintain the health of the wife or mother. Small signs of attention, a kiss goodbye, a bunch of wild flowers as a gift will make her day happy.

In Cancer women, the lymphatic system, breast, endocrine system, skin, mucous membranes are vulnerable. The most endangered are the female breasts, everything related to feeding the baby, the organs of the digestive system. A woman's health directly depends on the state of her nervous system. At any moment, an emotional lady can get seriously ill, but she will instantly recover from good news or a profitable deal. From the outside, it may seem that she is pretending to be sick in order to get her way. However, close people know that her health directly depends on her mood. Cancers are sincere and responsible people who simply try to choose the right moment in order to achieve their goals with the least loss.

## Good and bad habits

The most unstable and weak in nature Cancers are not able to withstand the circumstances, they are often prone to phobias, depression. Fears and excessive loads, an unfavorable environment, unsolvable tasks and bad habits can cause withdrawal into oneself, lead to the path of alcohol, narcotic and psychotropic substance abuse. It is almost impossible to return Cancer to real life, you need to spend a lot of energy, love and care for treatment and rehabilitation. Fortunately, abuse is rare. Cancers are distinguished by a great sense of responsibility, they cannot leave loved ones without care, forget about their duties.

Taking into account the peculiarities of the sign and the recommendations of the Cancer health horoscope, a sane representative of the element of Water can build his life in accordance with the rules of a healthy lifestyle. Proper nutrition, daily walks, morning exercises, fitness and sports will help to overcome the adverse influences of the planets, will enable Cancers to live a long and fruitful life. An important place in organizing a healthy lifestyle is taken by a positively minded family, a kind and sincere atmosphere at work, comfort and good friendships. Communication with relatives and friends has a beneficial effect on health. And good habits and a positive environment will save you from ailments and harmful influences.

## *Diseases and dangers, vulnerabilities*

According to the health horoscope, Cancers are vulnerable to injury and disease. People of this zodiac sign need constant monitoring of their health, regular supervision of doctors. From infancy, they carry all possible childhood illnesses. It should be borne in mind that little Cancer is experiencing hard discord and quarrels in the family, a poor emotional state of the child will immediately lead to illness or a nervous breakdown. In addition, children do not tolerate physical trauma well, they are sensitive to pain, and wounds and scratches take a long time to heal.

Adult representatives of the water sign are also very suspicious, easily panic-stricken, making "an elephant out of a fly." This feature often leads to more serious illnesses. Cancers need to take care of the head, brain vessels, lymphatic and endocrine systems, and the gastrointestinal tract. People of this sign are especially susceptible to chronic diseases: gastritis, peptic ulcer disease, pancreatitis, chronic constipation, diabetes mellitus, diseases of the nervous system. These diseases are especially exacerbated after 40 years, and can be dangerous if not kept under control. Literally all systems of the Cancer body do not work at full strength, if you do not help their work with a healthy diet, movement in the fresh air, and exercise.

# *Diet recommendations*

The diet for such a sensitive zodiac sign as Cancer must be balanced and carefully considered. Meals should not be overloaded with heavy meals, lots of meat. Protein needs are best met by eating lean poultry, seafood and fish. It is necessary to limit the use of salt, since the liquid in the body of Cancers often stagnates, the kidneys are not working actively enough. You should not get carried away with dough products and sweets, the body is not able to cope with a large amount of fast carbohydrates. At the same time, slow carbohydrates in the form of cereals, cereals will be beneficial. Vegetables, greens are necessary in the diet of a representative of the water sign, they help to remove undigested food and harmful toxins from the body.

We must not forget about the environment in which this sign feeds. Comfortable conditions, family atmosphere, friendly conversation will help the correct digestion process. Quarrels, unkind statements, negative emotions while eating are contraindicated for Cancers, they can cause a disease of the digestive system or a nervous breakdown. People of this sign are very vulnerable and require a special attitude towards themselves.

*Fitness and sports, outdoor activities*

Given the fitness horoscope, Cancers need to constantly monitor their health. These are fitness classes under the guidance of an experienced trainer without overloading. Morning exercises, light jogging in the fresh air, sea bathing are beneficial for a weakened body. It is also necessary to observe the regime of the day, work and rest. You shouldn't sleep too long, but you need to get enough sleep. Water procedures, swimming are the most useful activities for this sign.

Travel, tourism does not attract these couch potatoes too much, but walks in the fresh air, light exercise are very useful. Although family gatherings, household chores bring Cancers much more joy. Working in the garden can be of benefit and great pleasure to people of the water element. Communication with flowers, plants and animals will also please.

## *How to maintain and improve health*

In general, it is possible to preserve and strengthen the health of this unusual zodiac sign, but it requires serious efforts and careful attention. Observation and periodic examinations of a doctor are indispensable. A medical examination should be carried out annually to prevent the development of chronic diseases. A daily routine, a correct diet that does not allow excess weight, regular exercise and walking in the fresh air, swimming are useful to any person, but they are simply necessary for Cancer.

The representative of this zodiac sign should find a job, something to their liking, in which you can achieve success, material well-being. Cancer is a purposeful and hardworking person, capable of providing well-being, comfortable living for his family and children. The marriage should be strong, for life, and loved ones will provide comfort and support in any difficult situation. With the care of family and self-discipline, Cancer's life can be long and happy. In addition, art, music, contemplation of beautiful works of painting, visiting theaters, concerts are beneficial for the talented sign. Enjoying art, realizing their natural talents, Cancer gets a boost of energy and health.

# HEALTH HOROSCOPE: LEO

People born under the sign of Leo have a tremendous amount of energy. They have had excellent health since childhood. Leos can boast of excellent immunity, thanks to which they are not afraid of many diseases. Representatives of this sign are incredibly hardy and resilient individuals who are able to survive the blows of fate and stressful situations. However, representatives of the element of fire do not know how to correctly calculate their strength. They can plunge headlong into the work process, forgetting about rest and sleep, which naturally affects the state of their body. Leos try not to show weakness and do not like to talk about their diseases. They carry most of the diseases "on their feet" without seeking the help of doctors. Because of this, many ailments remain untreated and can manifest themselves at any time.

## *Leo man health horoscope*

Leo men are the owners of good health. They have a high resistance to various infections, as a result of which they are not afraid of colds. In case of illness, their body quickly recovers without any serious consequences. The health horoscope for Leos speaks of the love of this sign for sports and physical activity. Leo men never flaunt their weaknesses and try to get rid of the disease that torments them as quickly as possible. Representatives of the fiery element hate being inactive and never stop there.

Despite excellent health, Leo men often misjudge their capabilities, placing more on their shoulders than they can actually bear. Increased self-confidence often plays a cruel joke with them. In the hope that the problem will disappear by itself, representatives of this sign do not seek help from doctors for a long time. As a result, the disease remains with them for a long time and can manifest itself at the most inopportune moment. Leo men often suffer from fever, but they are not afraid of chronic diseases.

People born under this sign love to enjoy life and get the most out of it. With age, they may have extra pounds and a tendency to abuse alcohol. Bad habits can affect the state of the digestive system, heart and blood vessels. For Leo men, problems with the spine are characteristic. Astrologers recommend that they monitor their posture from childhood, and in adulthood, avoid lifting weights. Representatives of the fire sign often suffer from diseases such as tachycardia, ischemia, arrhythmia and atherosclerosis.

## *Leo woman health horoscope*

Leo women are people with excellent health. Diseases overtake them very rarely and at the same time quickly recede. Representatives of this sign are strong personalities who do not stop and do not retreat in front of difficulties. Energy in them is in full swing. However, they often work beyond measure, completely sparing themselves. Leo women never show their weaknesses, from which they can suffer from overwork and depression. In fact, these are vulnerable people, the best medicine for whom will be support from family and friends.

The most vulnerable organs in representatives of the fire element are the heart and blood vessels. Leo women are more likely to suffer from diseases such as thrombophlebitis, embolism, hemorrhage and heart attack. Often, diseases have an acute course, together with high fever. Astrologers recommend that the representatives of this sign rely on traditional medicine and not neglect medicinal herbs. Soothing decoctions will help overcome depression and relieve fatigue.

The Leos health horoscope warns women born under this sign to avoid overeating. They tend to be overweight and have problems with the gastrointestinal tract. Regular exercise can help you maintain your weight. It is recommended not to abuse, but it is better to completely abandon alcoholic beverages because of the danger of acquiring alcohol dependence. Do not forget about the back and bones, which are often injured and bruised.

## Good and bad habits

Despite excellent health, the horoscope advises Leo to develop a positive habit from an early age to monitor and maintain the state of their body at the proper level. Representatives of this sign are strong and self-confident individuals. They are distinguished by great intellectual abilities and strong-willed character. They are born leaders. At the same time, overconfidence can negatively affect their health. Leos often take on heightened commitments that they cannot always handle. They should not get involved in gambling, otherwise Leos risk being left with nothing.

People born under the sign of the fire element are extremely susceptible to flattery. Often, representatives of this sign are not able to distinguish real friends from hypocritical enemies. Among the most dangerous and most common bad habits of Leos, it is necessary to note the passion for alcoholic drinks and tobacco products. However, if they have a desire to defeat these addictions, Leos can do it with ease. In addition, people born under this sign are advised to reduce the number of calories they consume and not eat sweets. Excessive enthusiasm for flour products often leads to a set of extra pounds and even obesity, which will be extremely difficult to cope with.

## *Diseases and dangers, vulnerabilities*

The main danger to people born under the sign of Leo is fatigue and nervous strain. Due to a lack of vitality, the cardiovascular system often suffers. In this regard, the most common diseases in representatives of this sign are tachycardia, angina pectoris, atherosclerosis, aneurysm and other ailments associated with the activity of the heart muscle. In addition, people belonging to the fire element have a predisposition to fevers, fainting, blindness and other eye diseases. They often have a sore back, suffer from posture problems and complain of fragile bones that break under the influence of any injury.

Among the common diseases of Leos, nervous ailments can be noted. They are characterized by a depressive state associated with the awareness of the limitations of their capabilities. Problems with excess weight and the general condition of the gastro-intestinal tract are considered commonplace for them. Obesity affects the quality of their life, shortness of breath, nausea and recurrent pain in the chest area appear. Among other things, people born under the sign of Leo have an increased risk of developing meningitis, measles and rheumatism. Due to the fact that they perceive the disease as a challenge to their own strengths, Leos do not heed the advice of doctors and stop treatment as soon as the first improvements are outlined. The health horoscope recommends waiting for full recovery, otherwise unpleasant complications await Leos.

## *Diet recommendations*

A complete vegetarian diet is contraindicated for Lions. Their diet must include meat dishes. Veal, chicken, turkey and various seafood will bring the greatest health benefits. However, it is better to refuse fatty and smoked ones, since they provoke an increase in cholesterol levels and do not have the best effect on the work of the heart and stomach. Leos should not ignore vegetables and fruits when drawing up a menu. They are especially useful in old age. The diet must include onions, cucumbers, lemons, dried apricots, raisins, apples, figs and walnuts.

Astrologers advise eating a varied and easily digestible diet. It is important that the menu contains foods high in vitamins E and C, for example, sprouted wheat, lettuce, oranges, strawberries, watermelon, rose hips. It is important for representatives of this sign to monitor their weight and in no case should they abuse foods with a high sugar content. Among alcoholic beverages, it is better to give preference to red wine, which has a positive effect on the level of hemoglobin in the blood.

## *Fitness and sports, outdoor activities*

Leos are active people who love to prove their superiority. They seem to contain a source of endless energy. However, despite this, representatives of this sign are often lazy. Therefore, in order to achieve success in sports, they need to be selflessly involved and engaged from an early age. Fitness horoscope for Leos advises to give preference to those sports disciplines in which they can reveal their full potential.

It is important for people born under this sign to feel in the spotlight. They will show themselves in the best way in such sports as figure skating, gymnastics, skiing, golf. Variety dancing and fencing will be a good choice for them. People born under the sign of Leo make excellent football and hockey players. They feel great in extreme sports such as skiing, snowboarding and various types of wrestling. Representatives of the fire element often suffer from cardiovascular diseases. Cycling, aerobics, and regular jogging are suitable for strengthening the heart muscle.

## *How to maintain and improve health*

To maintain good health for many years, people born under the sign of Leo need to learn to relax and not take responsibility for everything in the world. Stress and overwork are their main enemies, which affect the functioning of the heart and blood vessels and negatively affect the state of the nervous system. Leos will benefit from moderate exercise. Daily walks in the fresh air will have a positive effect on their health.

In addition to stress, overeating and abuse of bad habits are dangerous for Lions. Representatives of the fire element are prone to a quick set of extra pounds, which will later be difficult to get rid of. People born under this sign are advised to reduce the amount of sugar they consume. The first symptoms that signal that it is time to change the diet and lifestyle are frequent shortness of breath, drowsiness and from time to time a pain in the chest that makes itself felt. In addition, a good 8-hour sleep is an important factor that will help maintain good health.

# HEALTH HOROSCOPE: VIRGO

Virgo is one of the most difficult signs in astrology. People born under this sign are obsessed with their health. This often turns out to be harmful to them, since Virgos find diseases even where they are not. They are hypochondriacs by nature. Representatives of the elements of the earth approach the choice of a doctor with great seriousness. They must learn all his ins and outs before entrusting him with their health. Thanks to a rational approach, Virgos live much longer than other signs, and older representatives of the sign do not experience serious health problems. Virgos have the nature of workaholics. They rest little and prefer not to sit in one place. In this regard, they often have problems with the nervous system. They suffer from overwork and insomnia. These are petty people, with a pessimistic outlook on life, who like to criticize others.

## *Virgo man health horoscope*

Virgo men are distinguished by good health and strong immunity. Since childhood, they have developed the habit of monitoring the state of their body, maintaining physical fitness, tempering and listening to the advice of doctors. Due to increased suspiciousness, men born under this sign tend to look for non-existent diseases in themselves and sound the alarm for the most insignificant reasons. At home they will certainly have medicines for almost all ailments. In some cases, their desire for perfection is brought to the point of absurdity, which is why Virgos begin to go to the hospital because of the slightest problems and try to follow the recommendations of doctors with all scrupulousness.

The most vulnerable places in the Virgo's body are the digestive system, spleen, gallbladder, pancreas and nervous system. Men born under this sign should especially beware of diseases such as gastritis, intestinal obstruction, stomach ulcers, hernia, appendicitis and colitis. In childhood, they may have helminths, and in adulthood, Virgos often suffer from intestinal disorders. They are characterized by various neuralgias and memory disorders. Often Virgo men suffer from all kinds of phobias and psychoses.

In most cases, diseases in representatives of this sign do not manifest themselves in any way, which seriously complicates their diagnosis. To maintain vigor and good mood, the health horoscope for Virgo advises you to learn to relax and not neglect your daytime sleep. It is important for people born under this sign to maintain peace of mind. Various hobbies, collecting and daily walks can contribute to this. In addition, Virgo men are not recommended to abuse sweet and flour products due to the existing tendency to obesity and the development of diabetes.

## *Virgo woman health horoscope*

For a Virgo woman, her health comes first. In most cases, they have excellent immunity and rarely suffer from various diseases. This is due to their passion for a healthy lifestyle. Representatives of this sign try to keep themselves in good physical shape in all situations, do not abuse alcoholic beverages and adhere to a healthy diet. However, they may be haunted by disturbing thoughts about the state of the body. It can be incredibly difficult to live with such people, as they impose their lifestyle on others.

Constant concern about one's own and someone else's health results in chronic nervousness and insomnia. Excessive stress negatively affects the state of the cardiovascular system. Overwork can cause chronic migraines. In addition, Virgo women often pay increased attention to hygiene. Over time, this hobby can develop into a real mania, which only a psychologist can help to cope with. The Virgo health horoscope advises them to relax more often and learn to rest.

The most problematic place in the body of a Virgo woman is the stomach. Often, representatives of this sign suffer from colitis, gastritis, constipation, appendicitis, dysentery, indigestion and other diseases of the digestive system. Correct, balanced nutrition will help Virgo to regain great health. Women born under this sign are not advised to abuse oily and spicy foods due to the increased chance of stomach ulcers. In addition, they have a tendency to gain excess weight.

## *Good and bad habits*

Virgos are perfectionists. They always get things done. The main thing for them is their own health. Outwardly, the representatives of this sign give the impression of a strong person, however, in fact, inside they are overwhelmed with emotions. Virgos never shy away from the task at hand and are determined and hardworking by nature. People born under this sign have a pathological tendency to maintain cleanliness. They are fair and do not like to stop there. If their dreams and aspirations are unfulfilled, Virgos will feel depressed and unhappy for a long time.

The most common bad habits of Virgins include the abuse of sweets and increased cravings for tobacco products. They need to avoid overeating due to their increased tendency to be overweight. They are indifferent to alcoholic beverages. Virgo and the day can not live without criticism of others. One of the most unpleasant habits of this sign is nit-picking. With their remarks, they spoil life and nerves not only for themselves, but also for loved ones. Increased anxiety about every issue can provoke a serious nervous breakdown, which they cannot get rid of on their own.

## Diseases and dangers, vulnerabilities

Virgo has the best health of any zodiac sign. This is not surprising, since its representatives tirelessly monitor the slightest deviations in well-being. With an insignificant sign of illness, people born with this sign immediately run to the doctor. Sometimes this attitude towards health can reach fanaticism, which in turn also provokes some deviations in health. Due to the large number of medications used, Virgos can develop serious allergies. Representatives of this sign suffer from frequent migraines, thyroid diseases and ailments associated with the respiratory system. Although it is worth noting that infections and colds are of little concern to Virgos.

As the health horoscope for this sign notes, the most problematic organs in Virgo are the digestive and nervous systems. People born under this sign often suffer from diseases such as acute intestinal infection, constipation, diarrhea, appendicitis, hernia, enteritis, colitis and gastritis. Due to the pathological desire for perfection, Virgos are prone to nervous and mental disorders. In turn, anxiety about every occasion can provoke problems with the cardiovascular system.

## Diet recommendations

Virgos have a weak digestive system, so astrologers recommend that they make a choice in favor of a vegetarian diet, in which, however, fermented milk products must be present. Kefir, yogurt, milk, soft cheeses have a positive effect on the stomach and normalize the intestinal microflora. The diet for Virgos should include plenty of pectin-rich fruits and vegetables. These include apples, beets, and carrots. They help to remove toxins from the

Virgo's body.

Representatives of this sign spend a lot of energy every day. You can replenish it from food that contains enough protein, such as eggs, fish, and lean veal. Foods such as wheat bran, chicory, almonds, zucchini and dates have a positive effect on the health of Virgins. Potassium sulfate plays an important role for the body of people born under this sign. It delivers oxygen to the cells. It can be found in oats, oranges, bananas, lemons, and wheat oil. Its deficiency leads to hair loss and brittle nails. Herbal tea will help to cope with indigestion, which Virgo often suffer from. It is better for them to refuse sweets, since there is a high chance of developing diabetes mellitus, as well as a tendency to fullness and rashes on the face.

## *Fitness and sports, outdoor activities*

Fitness horoscope for Virgo says that representatives of this sign can achieve great success in sports if they get used to physical activity from childhood. Natural modesty and isolation prevent them from realizing their potential in this field. Virgos are neat in everything. Sports are no exception. Mostly, people born under this sign perform various exercises only in order to maintain good physical shape for a long time.

Virgos are organized and can succeed in sports that require refined movements and coordination of their actions. The ideal disciplines for them would be figure skating, diving, mountaineering and sailing. It is useful for Virgos to strengthen the muscles of the abdominal cavity, which can be served by playing tennis, dancing and martial arts. In addition, intellectual games such as chess are suitable for these sophisticated natures.

## *How to maintain and improve health*

Virgo's digestive system is the weakest point in their body. Based on this, the horoscope recommends that representatives of this sign pay increased attention to the state of the intestines and stomach. Virgos are highly discouraged from abusing fatty, spicy and smoked food, as it can provoke the development of gastritis and stomach ulcers. People born under the sign of Virgo should not strain their abdominal muscles too much, however, you should not give up exercise completely. Exercising daily and walking in the fresh air will help maintain physical health for years to come.

Do not forget about the state of the nervous system. Regular rest will help keep your peace of mind. It is important for Virgos to learn how to relax, and not devote all their time to work. They need to acquire some kind of hobby or hobby. Virgos are encouraged to nap during the day to help them cope with constant stress and tension. The health benefits of this sign will bring mental activity, solving crosswords, puzzles, logic problems and even simple reading. Creative activities such as music or handicraft can help cope with stress.

# HEALTH HOROSCOPE: LIBRA

Unlike other zodiac signs, Libra has no mental health problems. They always strive for harmony, know how to rest for the benefit of their body and do not follow the lead of negative emotions. The health horoscope says that in most cases their problems are associated with excesses in food and bad habits, which they are completely unable to resist. Libra tries to avoid unnecessary physical exertion, since they do not have a large energy reserve. They do not like to be alone and prefer to spend most of their free time with friends. Left alone with their thoughts, Libra quickly becomes discouraged.

## *Libra man's health horoscope*

Libra men have a tendency to slow metabolism. This is a big problem for them due to their predisposition to overeating. In this way, representatives of this sign relieve internal stress. Astrologers recommend Libra not to overwork and learn to relieve internal discomfort. They cannot be alone for a long time, otherwise they are guaranteed to acquire a syndrome of a depressive state. Libra, like no one else, is important to develop a tendency to self-discipline. Various hobbies and daily morning walks will help them in this.

Men born under this sign often suffer from kidney disease. They have urolithiasis, uremia and diabetes, which also provokes rapid weight gain. Hypothermia is strictly contraindicated for Libra men due to a predisposition to viruses and infections. In addition, they should not lift weights, as there is a risk of ripping off their backs. Also, representatives of this sign are pursued by diseases of the gastrointestinal tract and allergies. Libra's circulation is not the best. They are constantly freezing, even in hot weather. In winter, they need to keep their limbs warm.

Often, Libra men are worried about the condition of the organs of vision and skin. The slightest discomfort will certainly affect the condition of the skin. Various rashes are common for them. They have absolutely no developed resistance to alcoholic beverages. Weak willpower leads to the fact that they quickly acquire alcohol dependence, which in the future will not be easy to get rid of. The health horoscope for Libra recommends developing an interest in sports from a young age if they want to maintain good health until old age.

## Libra woman health horoscope

Libra women always strive for harmony in everything, however, due to an overly active lifestyle, they do not always manage to achieve this. Representatives of this sign do not pay enough attention to their state of health. Many Libra women will seek medical help only in exceptional cases, when there is simply no other choice left. In the case of minor sores, they prefer to use folk remedies and rely solely on their own strength. The Libra health horoscope recommends listening more often to the state of the body, since many diseases are much easier to eradicate at the initial stage.

Women born under this sign cannot boast of strong immunity, which is why they are prone to colds. In the midst of infectious diseases, it is better for them to sit out at home. Increased attention should be paid to the genitourinary system and in no case should hypothermia be allowed. Libra women may suffer from increased bone fragility. Astrologers recommend avoiding traumatic situations and strengthening the skeletal system by eating foods with a high calcium content. Representatives of this sign are often worried about problems associated with the gastrointestinal tract and slowed metabolism. They are often overweight.

Libra women can suffer from insomnia and increased fatigue. The problem lies in their desire to always and everywhere be in time. They need to remember that the reserves of the body of any person have their limits. Libras are strongly encouraged to learn how to relax and not drive themselves into rigid frames. Regular rest will help them avoid dizziness and nervousness. In addition, regular walks in the fresh air and socializing with loved ones contribute to your well-being.

## *Good and bad habits*

Libra always gravitates towards the beautiful and harmonious. Representatives of this sign will never appear bad-looking in public. Their appearance is always perfect. Thanks to increased intuition, they manage to avoid serious illnesses. Libra has no predisposition to nicotine. Even starting to smoke, they will be able to quit this occupation at any time. Their natural desire for balance helps them perfectly control their emotions. Thanks to this quality, Libra almost never has a nervous breakdown.

Libra's bad habits include laziness and a propensity for uncontrollable waste. They are ready to come up with many excuses, just not to start performing their duties. People born under this sign of the air element often spend their savings on things they do not need. Libras also tend to seize their problems with sweets. Overeating, in turn, provokes a quick set of excess weight. Alcohol is also a great weakness of the representatives of this sign. Despite the lack of a natural propensity for alcoholism, Libra is in constant search of an alcoholic drink that will suit their taste. If their search is crowned with success, they will not avoid the appearance of alcohol dependence, from which it will be difficult to recover.

## Diseases and dangers, vulnerabilities

The weakest point in the Libra body is the kidneys and spine. Most of the serious diseases in representatives of this sign are associated with these organs. They often develop kidney stones and infections of the genitourinary system. It is dangerous for them to be exposed to hypothermia, since ailments of the upper respiratory tract are not uncommon for them. In old age, they themselves may experience diseases such as sciatica, lumbago, myositis and other ailments that appear in the lumbar region. The thighs, skin, organs of vision, the navel area are also considered weak points in the Libra's body, and the uterus is often affected by the female.

The nervous system is also exposed to various dangers. Excessive fatigue and increased stress can be factors affecting the onset of depressive syndrome and insomnia. Other diseases that the Libra horoscope warns about include skin rashes, tonsillitis, constipation, and glandular dysfunction. Regular migraines, which often signal more serious illnesses, can become a reason to see a doctor.

## Diet recommendations

Libra is a big food lover. Basically, they listen to the desires of their bodies, eating whatever they want. The Libra diet must necessarily contain a lot of fruits and vegetables. Astrologers recommend minimizing the consumption of fatty foods, and especially meat products. Libra often suffer from problems with the gastrointestinal tract, so it is undesirable for them to abuse flour products. Lean meat, mainly poultry and beef, sprouted wheat, vegetable oils, dairy products and various types of fish, will contribute to your Libra's well-being.

To prevent kidney failure, Libra is advised to add mineral salt rich in sodium phosphate to food. It normalizes the acid-base balance and promotes the removal of toxins from the body. Its lack leads to the development of apathy and a decline in vitality. For normal liver function, representatives of this sign need vitamin E, a large amount of which is found in foods such as alfalfa, malt and soybean oil. Dishes with iodine content are useful for Libra. Its sources are pumpkin and radish.

## Fitness and sports, outdoor activities

Sports and Libra are almost incompatible concepts. Representatives of this sign are not included in the list of exercise lovers. They are sophisticated natures who prefer art to exercise. At the same time, if desired, Libra can achieve significant heights in sports. Their main motivation for going to the gym regularly is admiring glances from the opposite sex. Fitness horoscope for Libra says that ballet or dancing will be the best sports for the female half of the sign. They can also play tennis, fencing, archery or basketball.

Libras have a strong sense of camaraderie, so they will feel great in team sports. Libra men, with the proper aspiration, will achieve great success in football or badminton. They will be able to excel in figure skating and alpine skiing. The main thing that guides people born under this zodiac sign is that sports should be fun. If this or that sports discipline ceases to bring them joy, Libra will immediately leave it. Representatives of this sign are contraindicated in extreme and dangerous sports, such as boxing or wrestling.

## How to maintain and improve health

The main enemy of Libra's health is hypothermia, which representatives of this sign should avoid by any means. In particular, it is worth protecting the lower back from it. Regular walks in the fresh air will help Libra to maintain good health until old age. Libra needs to learn how to rest in order to counteract nervous system problems. Constant overwork and poor sleep can lead to depression. People born under this sign don't like to be alone. To maintain excellent health, it is important for them to maintain communication with friends and family who can cheer them up during difficult times.

Weakened immunity is often the cause of infectious diseases. To increase its protective functions, Libra should strike a balance between periods of activity and inactivity. In no case should the representatives of this sign go to extremes, otherwise it will lead to depletion of the body. In addition, they should minimize the consumption of alcoholic beverages, otherwise it can lead to serious addiction.

# HEALTH HOROSCOPE: SCORPIO

People born under the sign of Scorpio have a high life potential from childhood. They are incredibly energetic and from the outside give the impression of an omnipotent personality. Often they cannot correctly calculate their strength, which goes sideways for them. Their self-confidence can lead to serious illnesses, from which Scorpios will suffer for a long time. They intuitively feel trouble and try to bypass them. Representatives of this sign are the owners of a rich inner world. It can be difficult to communicate with them because of their quick temper and self-centeredness.

## *Scorpio man health horoscope*

Scorpio men will be able to boast of good health right up to old age. They have a penchant for sports, which will play an important role in their well-being. At the same time, the health horoscope for Scorpios suggests that they will have a lot of difficult trials. They cannot imagine their life without risk and dangerous situations. Scorpios are prone to injury, various accidents and even car accidents are possible.

Representatives of this sign are often susceptible to viral and infectious diseases. They cannot resist them, therefore, during outbreaks of epidemics, Scorpios are not recommended to visit crowded places. In the fall and spring, they need to take as many preventive measures as possible. Despite this, illnesses proceed quickly and do not pose a serious danger to them. Scorpio men are prone to bad habits that can seriously undermine their well-being. The key to their health is moderation in all aspects of life.

For Scorpio men, urolithiasis, migraines, hepatitis, and caries are typical. They often suffer from problems with the stomach, digestive system, respiratory organs, kidneys, genitals, gall bladder and blood vessels. There are oncological diseases. Often, due to the inability to relax, the nervous system is in danger, there is a lack of sleep. An increase in physical activity will help the representatives of this sign get rid of nervous tension, especially if they lead a sedentary lifestyle.

## *Scorpio woman health horoscope*

Serious illnesses in Scorpio women occur only in childhood. Representatives of this sign have a huge amount of energy and an inexhaustible supply of strength. From the outside, it seems that there are no such problems that a Scorpio woman cannot cope with. They try to live life to the fullest and not deny themselves anything. Moderation is not characteristic of them. People born under this sign are prone to risky behavior, which often leads to numerous injuries that, fortunately, heal quickly.

The increased sexual activity of Scorpio women can cause sexually transmitted diseases. The genitourinary system and kidneys are their weak points. For them, infectious diseases are common and, if not properly treated, can become chronic. The Scorpio health horoscope advises them not to abuse alcohol and other bad habits, as they weaken their protective functions.

Scorpio women are often overweight, which in many cases is caused by the endocrine system. In addition, the representatives of this sign are haunted by diseases of the cardiovascular and respiratory systems, furunculosis, benign and malignant tumors, as well as ailments associated with the nervous system. Scorpio women are very emotional and do not tolerate criticism well. They know how to worry about any reason, as a result of which insomnia and increased fatigue occur.

## Good and bad habits

Scorpios are strong personalities with strong leadership qualities. They are incredibly purposeful and always get their way. Weakness is a vice for them. They do not like to talk about their problems to the people around them and try to cope with them on their own. Diseases try to heal on their own and rarely see a doctor. Thanks to their well-developed intuition, they sense an impending disease in advance and try to prevent its onset. Representatives of this sign hate flatterers. They directly express their complaints to the interlocutor. Despite the harsh statements, Scorpios are reliable and loyal friends. They will never tell someone else's secret.

Scorpios are secretive people. They rarely trust anyone. Failures can seriously undermine the emotional state of the representatives of this sign. Increased tension leads to problems with the nervous system, which in turn gives rise to the development of bad habits in Scorpios. In stressful situations, people born under this sign may start drinking alcohol, smoking, or seizing anxiety. They do not have a sense of proportion, so initially a slight hobby can quickly develop into a serious addiction, from which it will be difficult for Scorpios to get rid of. In such situations, they should not be alone. It is better for them to wait out a difficult period in the company of friends or close relatives.

## Diseases and dangers, vulnerabilities

People born under the sign of Scorpio are on the list of those who are trying to cope with the disease on their own without resorting to the help of doctors. Their diseases usually proceed extremely violently and quickly. Scorpio's health horoscope notes that one of the most vulnerable places in their body is the genitourinary system. Representatives of this sign are haunted by a whole list of diseases associated with it. They have: cystitis, urolithiasis, hemorrhoids, polyps, hepatitis, prostatitis and others. They often suffer from diseases of the kidneys, colon and small intestine, and bladder. In women, the uterus and ovaries are affected. Sexually transmitted diseases are often found in them.

Scorpio's vulnerabilities also include the cardiovascular system, blood vessels, respiratory system, digestive system, eyes and skin. Due to a slow metabolism, representatives of this sign may have difficulties with being overweight. The psycho-emotional side of Scorpios is also in danger. Increased activity and a desire to take everything into your own hands can lead to problems with sleep, fatigue and various kinds of ailments. People born under this sign should beware of infections and take preventive measures during epidemics. At such moments, astrologers do not recommend Scorpios to visit public places.

## *Diet recommendations*

Diet for Scorpions must contain protein foods. In their youth, they easily assimilate animal products: beef, pork, lamb, veal. Despite this, it is better to refuse it in old age, since problems associated with the health of the stomach and small intestine may occur. It is recommended to switch to lighter food. Scorpions benefit from fish and other marine animals. Fresh fruits and vegetables will be able to dilute the meat diet. Various vegetable salads and dishes from cereals have a positive effect on the digestive system of representatives of this sign.

The diet of Scorpions should include fermented milk products that promote the regeneration of intestinal microflora. Astrologers advise not to forget about prunes, figs, onions, cabbage, radishes, gooseberries and other dishes that contain calcium. It is essential for maintaining good skin condition, preventing the accumulation of toxins and increasing the overall immunity of the body. People born under this sign are extremely sensitive to the lack of vitamins C, E and B in the body. Products such as asparagus, radishes and plums can compensate for their lack. Scorpios are not recommended to overuse fatty and spicy foods, as this can lead to stomach ulcers, and also provoke obesity. Iron-rich foods will help to heal the body and improve immunity. These include: beef liver, buckwheat, nettle and black currant.

## Fitness and sports, outdoor activities

Fitness horoscope for Scorpio recommends that they give preference to active sports. Representatives of this sign cannot imagine their life without physical exertion. They are incredibly active and energetic people, accustomed to taking risks. They can achieve great success in a very short time. They will have a brilliant career in sports such as motorcycle and auto racing, running and bobsleigh. Extreme types of competitions are perfect for them, including mountaineering, cycling, triathlon and others. Scorpios excel in solo sports such as boxing and wrestling. However, if willing and with some effort, they can do well in team physical activities such as soccer or hockey.

The fair sex, born under the sign of Scorpio, thanks to their gracefulness and femininity, will achieve great success in synchronized swimming, dance, gymnastics and figure skating. Due to the weak genitourinary system, Scorpios should not choose sports related to heavy lifting and heavy load on the lower body. They are in no way recommended to engage in lifting and weightlifting. In addition, they need to avoid hypothermia in every possible way because of the danger of catching diseases associated with the respiratory system.

# *How to maintain and improve health*

Scorpios are incredible workaholics. The horoscope advises to rest more often, otherwise they will not be able to avoid over-work. It is this that is the worst enemy for the representatives of this sign. Scorpio should not ignore the alarming signals sent by their body. Representatives of this sign need to learn to be more moderate in all aspects of life, from food intake to intimate life. Fasting days will be able to prevent overeating, which are recommended for Scorpios every week.

Regular walks in the fresh air and giving up bad habits will help keep you healthy until old age. In general, a sedentary lifestyle is contraindicated for representatives of this sign. They must by any means maintain a high level of activity. Scorpios shouldn't be alone. Support from friends will help them avoid falling victim to depression and relieve depressed moods.

# HEALTH HOROSCOPE: SAGITTARIUS

Sagittarius is one of those signs who do not care about their health at all. They do not know the sense of proportion and often work for wear and tear. Excessive fatigue provokes illness and is the main reason for their poor health. In turn, poor sleep can lead to problems with being overweight and high blood pressure. Representatives of this sign are optimists in life. Thanks to their enormous life potential, Sagittarius quickly get rid of any disease. These are active people who are always at the center of events. They do not like to spend their free time alone and draw energy from communication with loved ones. Representatives of this sign are dependent on the opinions of others and easily succumb to other people's influence.

## *Sagittarius man health horoscope*

In most cases, Sagittarius men are in excellent health. However, a frivolous attitude towards your body can undermine it. Overwork and nervous tension play an important role in this. Representatives of this sign often do not spare themselves at work and do not sleep much. They can go headlong into their hobbies and not notice the signals that their body sends. In addition, nutrition has a great influence on their well-being. Since Sagittarius men are not big fans of a healthy diet, they may have problems with being overweight.

They should be wary of colds, especially tonsillitis. Astrologers advise avoiding visiting crowded places during epidemics and in no case forget about disease prevention. People born under the sign of Sagittarius should pay attention to the health of the spine, bones, stomach, and especially the liver. They should not abuse fatty foods and alcoholic beverages, as there is an increased risk of developing ulcers.

Sagittarius men are often clumsy. They are susceptible to various kinds of injuries, including when playing sports. They don't like going to doctors and staying in the hospital for a long time. Sagittarius will try to quit treatment as soon as possible, feeling even the slightest improvement in well-being. The Streltsov health horoscope says that representatives of this sign can easily live to a ripe old age if they take the state of their body with greater seriousness.

## *Sagittarius woman health horoscope*

Sagittarius women are attractive in appearance and have incredibly good health. In case of illness, they will postpone the visit to the doctor as far as possible, thereby bringing themselves to a critical state. Often they do not listen to the recommendations of specialists, so they think that they can take care of themselves. The representatives of this sign experience sudden mood swings, accompanied by a decline or rise in strength. Most often, Sagittarius women have problems with the respiratory tract and lungs. Colds are common for them.

The health horoscope for Sagittarius speaks of the possibility of diseases of the gastrointestinal tract, rheumatism, atherosclerosis and liver problems. Representatives of this sign should monitor their diet and try to eat healthy foods, as they tend to be overweight. Sagittarius women often suffer from overwork and lack of sleep, which makes them aggressive in communication.

Fatigue also affects the cardiovascular system and, in the worst case, leads to heart attack. Nervous strain leads to hypertension, the consequence of which can be a stroke.

Other problem areas for Sagittarius women include the lower limbs. For them, often such a disease as varicose veins. A sedentary lifestyle leads to it, to which the slopes of the fair sex in old age.

## Good and bad habits

Sagittarius is the soul of any company. These are incredibly sociable people who cannot imagine their life without friends and fun pastime. Representatives of this sign are amorous and are often torn between several partners. Sagittarius can do many things at the same time, which is often the reason for their increased fatigue and subsequent health problems. People born under this sign do not tolerate injustice and try to act according to their conscience in all situations. The negative sides of Sagittarius include excessive hot temper and impulsivity. They are often not in the mood and show aggression towards loved ones.

Representatives of this sign are dependent on the opinions of the people around them. They are subject to strong influence from outside. In most cases, Sagittarius acquire bad habits under the influence of the company. They may start drinking alcohol or smoking to stand out from the crowd and show their abilities. Over time, their bad habits develop into the strongest addictions, from which they cannot get rid of until the end of their lives. In addition, representatives of this sign are often unhappy with their lives. They often feel envy, which negatively affects the state of their nervous system.

## Diseases and dangers, vulnerabilities

Sagittarius can boast of excellent health by nature. Most of their well-being problems are caused by their own not being serious about him. They lead an active and hectic lifestyle that negatively affects the state of the body. The horoscope warns Sagittarius about such vulnerable places as the buttocks, thighs, liver and circulatory system. People born under this sign have a slow metabolism. It is important for them to follow a diet, as the stomach is one of the weakest organs in Sagittarius. Many diseases in representatives of this sign do not manifest themselves immediately, and for a long time they may not be diagnosed. Sagittarius have a serious predisposition to respiratory diseases. They often suffer from colds and pneumonia.

Astrologers warn of possible problems with the cardiovascular system, hip joints, as well as the colon and small intestine. In addition, Sagittarius complain of high blood pressure, which can lead to stroke in old age. Sagittarius often suffer from their clumsiness, leading to serious injury, dislocation and even bone fractures. They are not afraid of mental illnesses. They know how to switch their attention and not succumb to negative emotions. Along with this, excessive enthusiasm for any business can lead to increased fatigue.

## *Diet recommendations*

Sagittarius is an active sign, for which it is important to stay in good shape and always be ready to rush into battle. Protein food must be present in his diet. It includes: lean poultry, fish, dairy products, soybeans, beans, walnuts and seeds of various vegetables. In addition, the diet for Sagittarius must necessarily include dishes from vegetables and fruits. For the body of representatives of this sign, prunes, figs, strawberries, fresh salads, pears, apples, potatoes, green peppers and strawberries will be useful. All of these products are rich in silicon, which is essential for strengthening hair and maintaining healthy skin color. A deficiency can cause bleeding from the gums.

Astrologers recommend that Sagittarius give up fatty foods and refrain from drinking alcoholic beverages. Abuse of them negatively affects the condition of the stomach, which is a vulnerable organ in representatives of this sign. To maintain liver health, they advise reducing the amount of sugar you eat and focusing on foods that contain vitamins E, B4, and C. They can be found in cabbage, cucumbers, asparagus and oranges.

## *Fitness and sports, outdoor activities*

Sagittarius is an active sign that is usually fond of sports since childhood. Thanks to such traits of their character as hard work, patience and dedication, representatives of this sign easily reach great heights in any chosen discipline. In childhood, they can go to many sports sections at the same time, since it is difficult for them to give preference to one of them. They love to express themselves and demonstrate their abilities. Sagittarius has a high team spirit, so football, hockey, volleyball or basketball will be ideal sports disciplines for them. Athletics will also be able to reveal their natural potential well.

Sagittarius have a lot of stamina, which makes them great runners and cyclists. They show themselves quite well in motorsport. In addition, tennis, horse riding, swimming and luge are great for them. Sagittarius are not afraid to take risks, so extreme sports are also in their area of interest. Despite the increased physical activity, the fitness horoscope for Sagittarius speaks of their high abilities in intellectual competitions such as chess, checkers or fencing. People born under this sign do not have strong blood vessels and joints, therefore astrologers advise to refrain from weightlifting.

## *How to maintain and improve health*

The health horoscope advises Sagittarius to pay attention to prevention and pay more attention to their well-being. It is not recommended to bring the disease to a chronic state, as it will not be easy to get rid of it later. Astrologers recommend that representatives of this sign expose themselves to less dangers and avoid traumatic situations. An important part of maintaining health for Sagittarius is proper nutrition. A slow metabolism along with eating high-calorie foods can lead to extra pounds.

People born under this sign need more rest. Healthy sleep is a guarantee of excellent health and a positive attitude. Doing what they love and communicating with loved ones will help them get rid of nervous tension. Sagittarians shouldn't neglect outdoor walks. They will help not only strengthen blood vessels, but also relax well. In the midst of infections, representatives of this sign should avoid crowded places and take increased preventive measures. In the event of a cold, it is better for them to immediately seek help from a doctor before it takes on a chronic form.

# HEALTH HOROSCOPE: CAPRICORN

Capricorn is one of the signs that have difficulties with self-realization and health. Their state of health is directly dependent on age. In childhood, they are haunted by muscle weakness, and any disease often spills over into an acute form that is life threatening. Often illnesses acquire a chronic condition from which they suffer throughout their lives. In old age, representatives of this sign, on the contrary, are an example of vigor and excellent health. Distinctive features of Capricorns are incredible endurance and a well-developed instinct for self-preservation.

## Health horoscope for Capricorn man

The Capricorn man is a winner in life. He plans everything in advance and is always ready to rush into battle. Possesses an inexhaustible supply of strength and vitality. Representatives of this sign enthusiastically take on difficult tasks, as they see them as a great opportunity to demonstrate their abilities. The health horoscope for Capricorn says that men can boast of good health, despite the problems in childhood. They strictly follow the recommendations of doctors and try to notice the slightest changes in well-being.

In most cases, Capricorn men have joint and knee problems. Often they have a lack of calcium in the body, which makes the bones fragile and can break from the slightest injury. Also, a small amount of it has a negative effect on dental health. Capricorns must monitor the state of the cardiovascular and digestive systems. They are characterized by a slow metabolism, they need to take care of a balanced diet and in no case overeat. A serious danger to people born under the sign of Capricorn carries colds, which, if not treated, can cause pneumonia.

Doctors often diagnose depression in Capricorn men. A gloomy and depressed state is common for them. Representatives of this sign are worried about every little thing, which deprives them of energy and leads to nervous breakdowns. Capricorns often suffer from diseases of the lower extremities, arthrosis, arthritis, rheumatism, varicose veins and sciatica. Astrologers recommend getting out into nature more often and not neglecting physical exercises. They will help strengthen the Capricorn's immune system.

## Capricorn woman's health horoscope

Women born under the sign of Capricorn make great demands on both the people around them and themselves. They don't like surprises and often prefer careers over family. The health horoscope advises avoiding overwork, as it can cause depression and other diseases of the nervous system. Representatives of Capricorn, often suffer from insomnia. Astrologers do not recommend them to stay alone for a long time, as there is a high risk of becoming a recluse by old age.

In childhood, Capricorn girls do not get sick more often than others, but they have a tendency to allergies, dermatitis and skin rashes. They are often injured, but they have excellent immunity. They are not afraid of colds and viruses. The weak points of Capricorn women include the gastrointestinal tract. They are characterized by food poisoning, therefore astrologers recommend that they adhere to a diet from childhood and give preference to healthy food.

One of the vulnerable organs of Capricorns is the biliary tract. Avoiding spicy and fatty foods, as well as reducing the consumption of carbonated drinks, will help reduce the risk of problems with them. Other problem areas that women born under the sign of Capricorn should look out for include tendons, joints and bones. Often they do not notice the symptoms of a developing disease, as they are completely immersed in work. As a result, many diseases become chronic.

## Good and bad habits

Hard work can be attributed to both useful and bad habits of Capricorns. They always get the job done, but their over-zeal to get the job done as quickly and well as possible can lead to chronic fatigue. One of the main positive aspects of people born under this sign is determination. Capricorns will not act rashly. They are not subject to outside influence and will never go against their principles. Representatives of this sign easily transfer criticism to themselves and try not to be led by emotions. However, astrologers do not advise Capricorns to keep their feelings to themselves, as this can negatively affect the state of their nervous system.

People born under the sign of Capricorn are suspicious of the people around them. They are rarely the first to make contact with strangers and often have communication problems. Loneliness and inability to find a common language with people can cause alcohol addiction, which will subsequently be extremely difficult to get rid of. Capricorns definitely need a hobby to resist this addiction. They show a tendency to melancholy, often haunted by disturbing thoughts and fears for their future.

## Diseases and dangers, vulnerabilities

Representatives of this sign are difficult patients, since they all have their own point of view, and will not miss the opportunity to argue with the doctor. Often they do not notice the first symptoms of the disease, and the diagnosis will be checked several times. This attitude often leads to serious complications, as a result of which treatment can be delayed for a long time. In most cases, hypothermia, impaired blood circulation, as well as a lack of nutrients and vitamins lead to Capricorn diseases. In childhood, they are often injured.

The most vulnerable and painful places and organs of Capricorns include: knees, lower thighs, shins, bones and teeth. Most often, people born under this sign suffer from arthritis, arthrosis, salt deposits, atrophies, paralysis, nervous disorders and problems with the digestive system. The horoscope recommends Capricorns to seek help from specialists in a timely manner, otherwise a seemingly insignificant sore can develop into a serious and intractable disease. In addition, it is desirable for them to monitor the state of their thyroid gland, otherwise Capricorns risk acquiring metabolic problems.

## *Diet recommendations*

The diet for Capricorns must contain foods rich in protein and calcium. Calcium phosphate forms bone tissue, which is especially necessary for the representatives of this sign due to weak bones. A deficiency in it leads to joint pain, tooth decay and curvature of the spine. Calcium can be found in high amounts in foods such as orange, lemon, celery, spinach, broccoli, corn, peas, walnuts, and potatoes. Capricorn's diet should be varied and balanced, containing fruits, vegetables and cereals. Capricorns have an urgent need for vitamins D and P. The first is necessary for better absorption of calcium, and the second strengthens the walls of blood vessels. They can be found in egg yolk, butter, rose hips, onions, cranberries, and lingonberries.

Due to their lifestyle, it is difficult for representatives of this sign to eat on a schedule. This leads to the fact that they are either undernourished or eat too much food in one meal. In no case should they abuse spicy and fatty foods because of the increased likelihood of stomach ulcers. Lean, lean meat, such as veal, turkey or rabbit, can be a source of protein for them. You can also get the protein you need from seafood. Astrologers advise to give preference to trout, cod, perch, ruff, bream and pike.

## Fitness and sports, outdoor activities

Capricorns have shown an interest in physical activity since childhood. They are quite ambitious and boast excellent endurance. In this regard, the fitness horoscope for Capricorns says that, if they wish, they can achieve success in any sport. Volleyball, basketball and athletics are great for them. Thanks to their dedication, they do well in marathons. Often among the representatives of this sign there are biathletes and skaters. Capricorns are incredibly patient and can go to their first sports victory for many years. People born under this sign do well in water sports as well. They prefer swimming, rowing and ski jumping.

Capricorns are not afraid to test their strength in extreme sports. They show a passion for rock climbing and cycling. They show their abilities well in team competitions such as hockey or football. However, any physical activity must be approached with caution, since due to weakened bones, they have an increased chance of injuring their knees. You should also beware of hypothermia of the lower extremities.

## How to maintain and improve health

The main source of problems, as the Capricorn health horoscope says, is depression. It can lead to anxious thoughts, headaches, cardiovascular, kidney and stomach problems. Representatives of this sign, like no one else, are important to maintain a positive attitude in any situation and not succumb to despondency. In no case should they be left alone. In addition, you do not need to be led by your bad habits. Frequent consumption of alcoholic beverages will only lead to serious addiction, but will not cure the true problems. It is important for Capricorns to find their place in life: get a job they love, do creativity and spend more time with friends.

The second, no less dangerous misfortune of Capricorns is overwork. It is important for people born under this sign to learn how to relax, and not devote all their free time to work. Capricorns have a tendency to hypothermia, due to which the lower limbs, and in particular the joints, often suffer. Astrologers recommend that they dress for the weather and sunbathe more often. Walking in the fresh air will benefit their immune system. One of the most important points in maintaining health is diet. It is advisable for representatives of this sign to adhere to a healthy diet and not to abuse fatty foods.

# HEALTH HOROSCOPE: AQUARIUS

Aquarius is a sign related to the element of air. Its representatives are creative and sensitive individuals. Diseases overtake them suddenly, although the causes of the sores accumulate for a long time. The health of Aquarius depends on his psycho-emotional state. Simply put, these are people of mood. In most cases, they suffer from nervous tension and problems with the circulatory system. People born under this sign rarely monitor their health and do not spend much time in the hospital. Often they quit treatment halfway through, as they quickly get bored of the monotony.

## *Aquarius man's health horoscope*

Aquarius men come across as open, sociable people. However, solitude is often preferred to the crowd. In childhood, they often get sick, not differing in strength and endurance. Colds and pneumonia are common for them. The situation changes dramatically with age. Aquarius men can boast of good health, which little can harm. But diagnosing a serious illness is extremely difficult.

The health horoscope speaks of the low stress resistance of Aquarius men. The slightest violation of the usual comfort can lead to numerous nervousness and panic attacks. Representatives of this sign are also distinguished by the habit of falling into despondency and despair. The anxiety of this sign can cause an increased enthusiasm for extreme entertainment, which entails various kinds of injuries. Emotional distress can lead to insomnia.

The weak point of Aquarius men is the legs. They often complain of muscle spasms, varicose veins, and swelling of the lower extremities. Astrologers recommend that they avoid professions associated with increased stress on their legs. Often times, Aquarius men suffer from migraines and vision problems. Representatives of this sign should also pay attention to the health of the cardiovascular and circulatory systems. Living in a temperate climate will positively affect their well-being.

## *Aquarius woman health horoscope*

Aquarius women are distinguished by high intellectual abilities and increased emotionality. They are artistic natures who love to be in the spotlight. Representatives of this sign strive to come to the aid of those in need as often as possible, which often does not benefit their health. Due to their high sense of responsibility and empathy, they suffer from insomnia, overwork and fatigue. Despite the emotionality, they do not like to show in public what is in their souls. Such secrecy negatively affects their health.

The horoscope advises Aquarius women to avoid overwork and rest more often. For chronic fatigue problems, they can benefit from exercise and outdoor exercise. Astrologers recommend paying attention to the condition of the heart, blood vessels and joints. In addition, the fair sex is prone to various kinds of allergic reactions and colds, up to chronic lung problems. It is important for them to carry out hardening procedures from childhood, to strengthen the immune system.

The unhealthy lifestyle and unhealthy diet can aggravate the painful condition. For representatives of the air element, it is important to follow a balanced diet that will help eliminate toxins from the body. In old age, Aquarius women have vision and lower limb problems. Often, women in years suffer from varicose veins and thrombosis. The health horoscope for Aquarius advises avoiding a sedentary lifestyle and do not forget to warm up for your legs.

## Good and bad habits

Aquarians cannot imagine their life without new experiences. Due to their light nature, they will always find an approach to any person. Their kindness and openness attracts new acquaintances. It is believed that representatives of this sign are the best advisers and can find a way out of any difficult situation. At the same time, Aquarians themselves rarely accept help from outside. People born under this sign are extremely freedom-loving and not influenced by outsiders. There can be no authority for them. Aquarians have a large supply of vital energy, thanks to which they easily cope with the blows of fate. They are not vindictive and quickly forgive insults.

Speaking about negative traits and bad habits of Aquarius, one cannot fail to note their overestimated self-esteem. These people do not like to wait and are not a model of patience. They will not dissemble and speak in riddles, as a result of which they can unintentionally injure the interlocutor with their words. Aquarians are prone to alcohol and nicotine addiction, which will be very difficult for them to get rid of. An increased desire for freedom and independence over time has a chance to develop into a mania that scares off friends. The best solution for Aquarius will be to translate their nervousness into a creative channel.

## Diseases and dangers, vulnerabilities

The most vulnerable places in the body of Aquarius are the lower limbs, in particular the calves and ankles. Ligaments, vessels, tendons, organs of vision, and the nervous system are also considered weak points. Doctors note they have a predisposition to kidney disease, pneumonia, allergies and a tendency to various injuries. The provoking factor of many physical disorders is increased fatigue and fatigue, leading to a weakening of the immune system. The result can be the onset of a depressive syndrome.

Commonly diagnosed diseases in Aquarius are cataracts and varicose veins. Astrologers noticed that cataracts develop in those representatives of this sign who strive to be in time everywhere, and try to take everything from life. Varicose veins persecute those who devote a lot of time to sedentary work. Problems often do not manifest themselves for a long time. However, if they were found to get rid of them is difficult, and their course is quite severe. Aquarians acquire a large number of disorders due to a neglect of their own health.

## Diet recommendations

People born under the sign of Aquarius are not particularly demanding for food. They are used to enjoying life and can find pluses even in the simplest dishes. Aquarians are in dire need of the presence of vitamins C and E in the foods they eat. This is due to a weakened circulatory system, which they help to strengthen. They can be found in apples, lemons, grapes, pears, oranges, and pineapples. Products containing a large amount of calcium will help get rid of nervous disorders: milk, kefir, soybeans and almonds. It is advisable for representatives of this sign not to abuse animal fats. Meat dishes should not be central to their menu.

The diet for Aquarius should be mostly vegetarian. It is useful for them to eat foods that do not need heat treatment. The diet of this sign should include seafood, in particular ocean fish and seaweed. Eating various vegetables, such as tomatoes, carrots, pumpkin, asparagus, radishes, spinach, as well as cereals, has a positive effect on the state of the body and maintains it in good shape. Astrologers advise Aquarius to arrange periodic hunger strikes and cleansing the body of toxins. This will help reduce the likelihood of health problems in old age.

## Fitness and sports, outdoor activities

Aquarians are freedom-loving personalities who are great at extreme sports. They are constantly in search of new experiences and quickly cool down in relation to this or that hobby. Thanks to their lightning-fast reaction, people born under this sign will become great basketball players. They can also achieve great success in athletics. Aquarius is a sign of air, so it is not surprising that its representatives are drawn to sports activities associated with this element. Fitness horoscope for Aquarius advises them to try themselves in parachuting. These people do well in mountaineering, cross-country skiing and figure skating.

Aquarians are not used to restrictions, so it is important for them to unleash their creativity, even in sports. Dancing and parkour will be the ideal solution for such individuals. They have a good attitude towards excursions and will not refuse to hike through caves, rocks or dense forests. Older sign representatives will enthusiastically accept mystical and spiritual practices, such as yoga. However, they will not be enough for a long time due to the overflowing energy from within and the inability to sit in one place. Due to their well-developed communication skills and the ability to find a common language with people, Aquarius can enjoy team sports, such as football or hockey, especially if they will occupy a leading position in the group.

## How to maintain and improve health

In order to maintain good health, the Aquarius health horoscope advises avoiding stress and nervous overstrain. It is extremely important for people born under this sign to find a hobby that can distract them from everyday problems and get away from reality for a while. Aquarians, no matter how they want, should not keep all emotions in themselves and hide them from others. A timely release of accumulated feelings will also help them maintain peace of mind. Astrologers recommend revising your social circle and, if possible, excluding from it people who annoy them and make them experience negative emotions. Decoctions and tinctures of medicinal herbs, such as chamomile, will help Aquarius to soothe shattered nerves.

The body of Aquarius is beneficially influenced by regular hardening and physical activity. Daily morning and evening runs, as well as fresh air, will charge them with a sense of vigor for the whole day. To avoid problems with varicose veins, regular water procedures, for example, going to the pool or relaxing on the seashore, will allow. In addition, you need to exclude long standing on your feet. Astrologers recommend monitoring your diet and not allowing excess nutrition, as Aquarius is prone to rapid weight gain. To maintain health until old age, it is important to stop drinking alcohol and smoking tobacco. Also, don't forget about healthy and regular sleep.

# HEALTH HOROSCOPE: PISCES

Pisces is a sign representing the water element and completing the astral cycle. According to astrologers, people born under his auspices do not shine with good health. Usually these are suspicious individuals who are in constant search for non-existent diseases. They are distinguished by kindness, which in most cases does not benefit them. Their good nature is used by manipulators, drawing Pisces into adventurous events. The main enemy of their health is the stress that they can experience for any reason.

## *Pisces man's health horoscope*

Males born under the sign of Pisces treat their health with great care. They can pinpoint an impending disease with incredible accuracy by its first signs. In old age, it can even develop into an obsessive state. The health horoscope for male Pisces recommends that they pay attention to the respiratory system and the gastro-intestinal tract. Pisces men are prone to colds and often suffer from vision problems. They have mood swings and increased fatigue. The best solution is to adhere to the daily regimen and healthy sleep.

It is worth paying attention to the health of the lower limbs. Pisces men are at high risk of developing fungal diseases, injuries and fractures. Representatives of this sign more often than others develop nerves and other mental illnesses. Alcoholic drinks and narcotic substances are especially dangerous for them. In them,

Pisces are looking for a way to escape from reality and their own failures. But their frequent use can lead to the development of serious addiction. In addition, men born under the sign of Pisces quickly get used to various medications, and therefore, conventional methods of treatment may not work on them.

Despite all of the above, among the male Pisces there are many vegetarians and people who lead a healthy lifestyle. The most effective means for maintaining immunity are water procedures. Rest at the sea, as well as regular use of medicinal and aromatic baths can seriously improve their health. In addition, the horoscope advises not to abuse coffee, as it increases nervous excitement. Representatives of the sign born in the third decade have the greatest endurance and good health.

## *Pisces woman health horoscope*

Pisces women are not very healthy, which also affects their appearance. The fair sex is often the owner of a fragile physique, and the absence of subcutaneous fat gives them a slightly painful appearance. For the most part, women born under this sign are weak in character and subject to various kinds of manipulations. Many of them live in their imaginary world and give the impression of people cut off from reality. They are real dreamers who too keenly feel all the events and changes happening to them, which affects their well-being.

The health horoscope of Pisces warns of a serious likelihood of undergoing various diseases of the nervous system. In order to balance their inner world, they are advised not to neglect various spiritual practices such as yoga or qigong. Creative classes also have a beneficial effect on the nervous system. It is important for Pisces women to have a job they love, otherwise they will feel unhappy. Boredom is contraindicated for them. You should not seek solace in various bad habits, since it will not be easy to get rid of them later.

Due to their increased susceptibility, Pisces women get sick much more often than other signs. Astrologers recommend spending more time on the health of the legs, lungs and vision, as these are the most vulnerable places in Pisces women. Due to belonging to the water element, rest on the sea coast will help improve the general condition of the body. Regular foot baths can help relieve tension and swelling in your feet. Eating a healthy diet is helpful. Eating all kinds of fruits and berries, as well as seaweed, has a positive effect on the female body and restores its tone.

## Good and bad habits

Traditionally, Pisces is considered the weakest sign of the zodiacal circle, however, and it is not devoid of some strengths. The most useful habit of people born under this sign is the ability to be in the right place at the right time. They have a well-developed intuition, which helps them to notice the first symptoms of an impending illness. From the outside, representatives of this sign seem weak and incapable of decisive action. However, they are often the first to come to the aid of those who need it. Other positive traits of Pisces include their sharp mind and well-developed intellectual abilities.

Pisces is a weak character, easily subject to various kinds of manipulations. The most dangerous bad habits of Pisces are alcohol and drug addiction. Due to the emerging depressive and melancholic state, they may look for a way out in a bottle. Representatives of this sign become a kind of vest for their friends and relatives. This, in turn, can negatively affect their mental health. Their reliability can lead to falling into bad company. Having become a victim of manipulation, they can decide on an illegal act.

Due to the weak willpower, Pisces are intemperate in food, which leads to overweight in old age.

## *Diseases and dangers, vulnerabilities*

Health for Pisces is the greatest value in life. Despite this, they are in no hurry to see a doctor in case of illness. In addition, a huge part of the ailments are just self-hypnosis due to increased nervousness. Representatives of this sign love to self-medicate and do not neglect folk methods. Any real disease is tolerated by people born under this sign rather hard, due to the initially not very strong state. They have weak immune systems, and worrying thoughts seriously slow down their recovery. Pisces has a slow metabolism, which increases the time it takes to remove toxins from the body. In this regard, they need to take various medications with increased caution, and only on the recommendations of doctors.

Based on the health horoscope, the most vulnerable and painful places in the body of Pisces are the lymphatic system, lungs, heart, gastrointestinal tract and lower limbs. Representatives of this sign are often prone to colds and fungal diseases. Diseases of the organs of vision, for example, conjunctivitis, are not uncommon. Their increased suspiciousness and melancholy leads to problems with the nervous system. People suffering from schizophrenia are found among the representatives of this sign with enviable regularity. In addition to the ailments listed above, many Pisces throughout their lives suffer from diseases of the legs, and in particular the feet. To reduce the severity of this problem, it is recommended that you wear extremely comfortable shoes.

## *Diet recommendations*

To improve their health, it is extremely important for Pisces to eat a balanced and healthy diet. A vegetarian diet for Pisces is the most optimal option, since their body has difficulty absorbing protein foods. The diet of Pisces must include such foods as lettuce, spinach, seaweed, cucumbers, beans, raisins and other fruits and vegetables. It is highly discouraged for fish to eat fatty foods. After them, they will feel heaviness in the stomach, become tired and irritable. The gastrointestinal tract is one of the most vulnerable places in the Pisces body. According to the recommendations of astrologers, young representatives of this sign can dilute their diet with lean turkey and chicken. Lean veal and beef liver won't hurt either. You should not give up fermented milk and fish products.

In the second half of life, it is better to give preference to plant foods. It is recommended not to neglect nuts, soybeans and grains. It is necessary to completely exclude alcoholic beverages from the menu, reduce the amount of sugar and various flour products. They disrupt the intestinal microflora and have a destructive effect on the body. A large amount of carbohydrates, which are usually found in sweets, contribute to the formation of mucus in the stomach, which slows down the already poor metabolism of Pisces. It is also desirable to reduce the amount of salt consumed. In large quantities, it leads to swelling of the legs.

## *Fitness and sports, outdoor activities*

Pisces is a sign of the water element, so it is not surprising that its representatives are drawn to sports related to water. Fitness horoscope for Pisces recommends that they pay attention to such sports activities as figure skating, synchronized swimming, rowing, sailing. Also, people born under these signs may like tennis and football. Astrologers do not recommend them to associate their lives with heavy and traumatic types of physical activity. They should give up sports such as wrestling or weightlifting.

You need to approach sports with caution, since legs are one of the weak points of Pisces. There is always a chance of joint dislocation or muscle strain. Daily walks in the fresh air and morning runs will help Pisces to maintain excellent health. Perfectly relieve tension, and increase muscle tone, yoga classes and various meditations. It is necessary not to overload your body during sports activities. Excessive passion for physical activity will only harm the health of Pisces.

## How to maintain and improve health

The most important condition for maintaining and strengthening the health of the body for representatives of this sign is to minimize the amount of stress received, since it is directly related to their emotional state. People born under the sign of the water element need to experience emotional upheavals as rarely as possible. They often overwork and experience a decline in vitality. To prevent this from happening, representatives of this sign need daily good rest. Pisces, like no one else, it is important to learn to love and accept themselves.

Regular massage of the lower extremities will not be superfluous. Legs are their sore spot, so you should monitor their health especially carefully, try to avoid hypothermia and all kinds of injuries. Water procedures strengthen health well. It is useful for fish to go on a trip to the sea at least once a year. The sea air has a positive effect on their well-being and perfectly strengthens the immune system. A good way to relax for Pisces is to engage in creativity, since by their nature they are dreamy people who spend a lot of time in their fantasies. Various stretching exercises also contribute to health. However, the most important thing for them is to learn to see the world in bright colors and look everywhere for positive moments.

# ABOUT THE AUTHOR

## Alex Magic

This amazing book was written by the great practicing feng shui master and astrologer of our time. The author is Professor of Psychology, Doctor of Astrology and Parapsychology of the London School of Astrology, Honorary Academician of the School of Traditional Medicine and Feng Shui Practice of China.
A successful astrologer of our time, author of textbooks and founder of the school of astrology and feng shui Alex Magic, where he teaches according to his own method, which has long established itself as the strongest and incredibly effective.